Introduction

Welcome to the next generation of pureed food! I created these recipes for anyone who needs to eat soft/blended food. I understand the frustration of seeing the same bland, unappetizing food on your plate day after day. You don't need to eat processed food from a can!

My recipes use fresh ingredients and whet your appetite with vibrant colors and enticing flavors and aromas. They are heart-healthy, simple and quick to prepare. Several do not even require a blender. Many are gluten-free, dairy-free and have no cholesterol.

To access more recipes and information on dysphagia, visit: www.dysphagiadietrecipes.com.

A special "Thank You" to Heather Boucher and Phil Cockfield who were both instrumental in helping me share these recipes with the online community.

Disclaimer

The author makes no representation that home preparation of these recipes is suitable for all individuals. The information presented is not intended to diagnose, treat or prevent any health related condition or to be a substitute for professional medical advice. Consult with your physician, dietician/nutritionist and/or speech-language pathologist for any questions or concerns regarding your individual diet needs, restrictions or texture modifications.

Think Outside the Blender

How to make great-tasting and healthy pureed food

- Spice it up with no-salt seasonings such as: garlic, lemon zest, thyme, turmeric, ginger, cumin or cinnamon - adjust to your taste.

- Look for foods that are naturally soft in texture like polenta, avocados and ricotta cheese.

- Potatoes, yams and various squashes (acorn, butternut) become very soft and easily mashed when baked - just add a little seasoning.

- Vary the temperature of foods, for example try gazpacho soup which is served chilled, as are fruit and yogurt smoothies; some fruits can easily be blended and frozen.

- Use a variety of colors on your plate, for instance top food with a bright red tomato sauce or a deep green pesto; or use baked yams instead of regular white potatoes.

- Experiment with food molds of various shapes and sizes to add height and interest to whatever food you are preparing.

- Canned beans such as cannellini, kidney, pinto and/or black beans - rinsed, drained and heated - are easily mashed and are a good source of protein with no cholesterol.

- Don't forget about presentation; take care to arrange food on the plate, add garnish (remove before eating) or use different colored dishware to make food look more appetizing.

Use these suggestions and your own imagination, have fun in your kitchen and

Think Outside the Blender!

For information regarding your individual diet needs, check with your doctor, registered dietician and/or speech-language pathologist.

Breakfast

Breakfast should be something you look forward to when you get up in the morning. There are many ways to incorporate fruit, yogurt and oatmeal into your breakfast meal. You will also find some non-traditional breakfast foods like yams and sweet potatoes - all healthy options to get your day off to a good start.

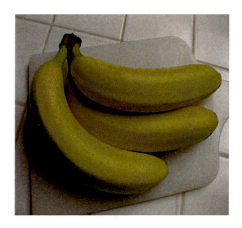

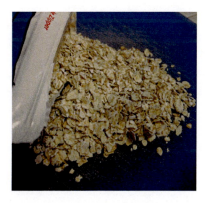

Strawberry Stacks

I love strawberries! Look for berries that are in season, organic and locally grown if possible.

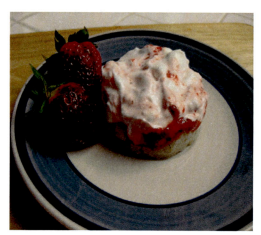

4-5 medium strawberries, stems removed and chopped

1/2 cup plain or vanilla yogurt (I find that Greek yogurt holds its shape well for this recipe)

1 serving of your favorite oatmeal

Make the oatmeal and let cool, set aside. Blend strawberries in blender/food processor until smooth (or use immersion blender). Fold blended strawberries into yogurt. Using a small, round food mold, place a few spoonfuls of oatmeal into bottom of mold and press down with spoon to make an even layer. Top with a few spoonfuls of yogurt/berry mixture. Carefully lift away mold and enjoy.

Apple Cinnamon Swirls

If you like the combination of apples and cinnamon, you'll love this! Check the applesauce label for gluten-free (or be adventurous and make your own – see recipe under Sides).

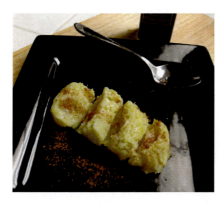

1 medium sweet potato, baked, cooled, peeled and mashed

1 tsp applesauce

light dusting of cinnamon

Spread room temperature mashed sweet potato onto parchment paper, creating a 4 inch by 6 inch rectangle with the longer side towards you, about 1/4 inch thick. Spread applesauce on top. Shake a little cinnamon on top of that. Lift up the long side of the rectangle and slowly start to roll it over, using a spatula to peel it away from the parchment paper. Move onto plate. Dust with a little more cinnamon. Slice and serve.

Maple Walnut Swirls

Another great-tasting recipe using simple ingredients. The walnuts and maple syrup are a wonderful flavor combination. Pure maple syrup is pretty strong (and has no corn syrup), so you only need a little bit.

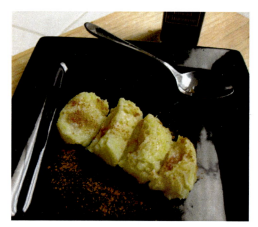

1 medium sweet potato, baked, cooled, peeled and mashed

1 tsp pure maple syrup

3 Tbsp walnuts, finely ground in food processor

Use the same method for laying out the mashed sweet potato as in previous recipe. This time, spread a layer of finely ground walnuts on top, followed by a drizzle of maple syrup. The pure maple syrup is very sweet, a little goes a long way. Lift the edge of the sweet potato rectangle up and over, carefully peeling away the parchment paper to create your roll. Move to plate. Drizzle with a little more syrup. Slice and serve.

Jammin' Oatmeal Bars

If you have a sweet-tooth like me, you'll love these! Use gluten-free oats if needed.

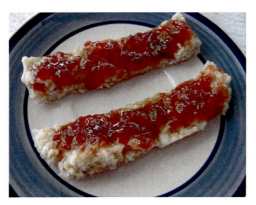

1 serving of your favorite oatmeal (cooked)

1-2 tsp your favorite jam (smooth)

Spread oatmeal evenly onto a small square dish (around 5"x5") or form into a square on a flat plate and allow it to come to room temperature. Cut into 4 equal bars. Top each with jam.

Cooking tip: quick oats are cut smaller than regular, rolled oats and will have a smoother texture when cooked.

Banana Yogurt Parfait

Little bites of pure bliss! Use the back of a fork to press through the banana. Ripe bananas work best.

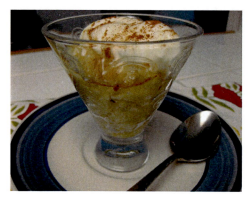

1 banana, peeled and mashed

plain yogurt

honey or agave

cinnamon

Layer banana then a spoonful of yogurt in parfait cup. Drizzle with honey or agave. Lightly dust with cinnamon.

Cooking tip: plain yogurt has much less sugar than fruit-flavored yogurt.

Oatmeal

Oatmeal doesn't have to be boring. With all the health benefits, it's worth taking another look. There are many ways to jazz it up to get your morning off to a good start. Personally, I like it with brown sugar and cinnamon, however, lately I've been adding applesauce, too. If you buy packaged rolled, quick or steel cut oats, follow the directions on the package. You can also buy oats in bulk which costs less and uses less packaging – better for you and the planet.

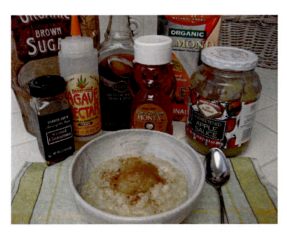

1/4 cup quick-oats

3/4 cup water

1/8 tsp salt – optional

Bring water and salt to a boil. Stir in oats and reduce heat to medium-low, cook 2-3 minutes, stirring occasionally, until all the liquid is absorbed. Add your favorite topping such as cinnamon, honey, agave nectar, brown sugar, applesauce, maple syrup, almond milk...Or swirl in a spoonful of your favorite jam.

Fruit & Yogurt Parfait

This is another refreshing treat. I always keep a bag of frozen berries in the freezer. Then they're available all year round.

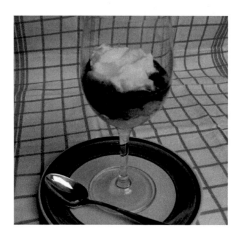

1/2 cup blueberries (or any other favorite berry), blended

1/4 cup plain yogurt

½ banana, mashed

Add a few spoonfuls of yogurt into glass and then a few spoonfuls of banana and blended berries; top with a dollop of yogurt.

Cooking tip: frozen berries work well too, just thaw and blend.

Strawberry French Toast

This really works -- the bread and berries soften a lot when cooked.

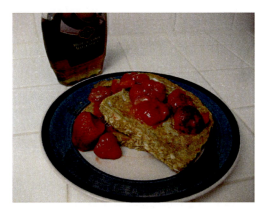

2 slices whole wheat bread, crusts removed

1 cup frozen strawberries

1 egg

1/4 cup almond milk

dash cinnamon

pure maple syrup

canola oil

Beat egg and add almond milk in shallow bowl, add cinnamon. Heat non-stick skillet lightly brushed with canola oil over medium heat. Dip bread slices one at a time into egg mixture, coating each side. Place each slice into skillet and cook 2-3 minutes on each side, until golden brown. In the meantime, cook strawberries in saucepan until the berries are warm enough so a fork can easily press through them (at this point you could blend the berries for a smoother texture). Add French Toast to plate; layer strawberries between pieces of toast and also on top. Drizzle with maple syrup.

Sweet Yam Pancakes

The flavor combination here reminds of autumn, but you can make these anytime.

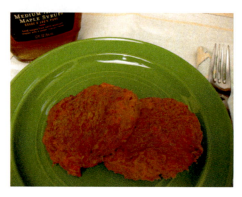

1 16 ounce yam, baked, cooled, peeled and mashed

1/4 cup flour

1/2 tsp grated ginger

1/8 tsp allspice

1 tsp brown sugar

1 Tbsp ground flax mixed with enough water to egg consistency

dash salt

pure maple syrup

Mix all ingredients, except maple syrup. Heat a little olive or canola oil in pan over medium heat. Drop batter by 1/4 cup into pan and cook 4-5 minutes per side. Drizzle with maple syrup. Makes 4 pancakes.

Smoothies

Use your imagination and any combination of fruit that you like for these smoothies. You can adjust the thickness by adding more or less liquid.

Cooking tip: an immersion blender makes it easy to whip up smoothies right in the glass.

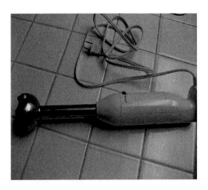

Tropical Smoothie

I like this one served chilled and I love the color! Great for breakfast or anytime.

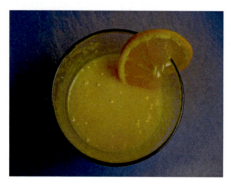

juice from one orange

1 cup frozen mango chunks, thawed

1/2 banana, cut in pieces

1/4 cup light coconut milk

1 tsp lime juice

Blend all ingredients.

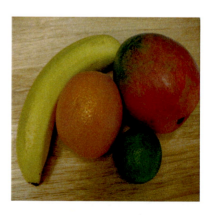

Fruit and Yogurt Smoothie

A great way to get more fruit into your diet. Also try coconut milk for a tropical flavor.

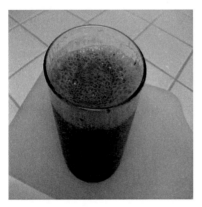

1/2 cup almond milk

1 small banana, cut into pieces

1/2 cup blueberries (or any other favorite berry) – frozen berries work well too

1/4 cup plain yogurt*

Add almond milk, then banana, berries and yogurt to blender (or to large cup if using an immersion blender). Blend until smooth.

* You could also omit the yogurt for a dairy free smoothie.

Pumpkin Pie Smoothie

I wish the photo conveyed the true pumpkin orange color of this smoothie – you'll have to try it and see for yourself. The texture is velvety smooth. If you like pumpkin pie, you'll love this!

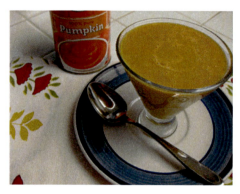

1/2 cup almond milk

1/4 cup pumpkin puree

2 spoonfuls of plain yogurt

1/2 tsp agave nectar

1/4 tsp cinnamon

light dusting of nutmeg and allspice

2 drops of vanilla extract

Pour all ingredients in blender and blend.

Lunch and Dinner

The variety of Lunch and Dinner items shows how food for dysphagia diets can be appetizing and taste great. Feel free to modify any of the spices/seasonings to suit your taste.   Many of the recipes are gluten-free and can be made dairy-free by omitting the cheese. Several types of beans and legumes are used as a good source of protein without adding cholesterol. Experiment with the cooking time for the polenta recipes. Polenta may become too crisp or hard to cut through if cooked too long, so reduce the time as needed.

Cooking tip: food molds are inexpensive and come in a variety of shapes and sizes. They can be found at kitchen supply stores.

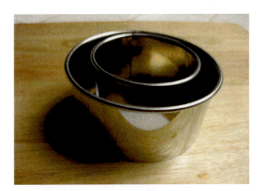

Naked Samosas

Samosas are little pastry pockets filled with spiced potato. They are "naked" here because we're only making the filling (no outer shell) which is very flavorful. Adjust the amount of seasonings to your taste. You can serve these with plain yogurt if you're ok with dairy.

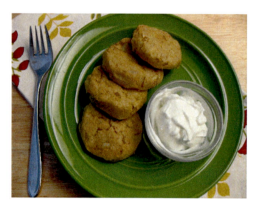

1 large russet potato, peeled and cubed

1 tsp olive oil

1/4 cup very finely chopped onion

1 clove garlic, minced

1 tsp freshly squeezed

lemon juice

1/2 tsp garam masala

1/4 tsp chili powder

Place potato cubes in pot and fill with water. Bring to a boil and boil for 10-12 minutes, drain and set aside (or you could use left over plain mashed potatoes). Heat olive oil in pan over medium heat. Add onions, then garlic and cook, for ~ 5 minutes. Add lemon juice, garam masala, chili powder and a pinch of salt and cook for 2-3 more minutes. Add in the cooked potatoes and mash well as you stir into onion mixture. Cook for 2-3 minutes until well incorporated. Set aside to cool. Preheat oven to 350 degrees. Form potato mixture into 2-3 inch rounds and place on baking sheet lined with parchment paper. Bake for 20 minutes.

Cooking tip: look for polenta in a tube and it's easy to cut into any shape you like.

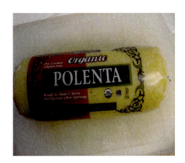

Polenta Tostada

Here's one way to use polenta if you've got a craving for Mexican food.

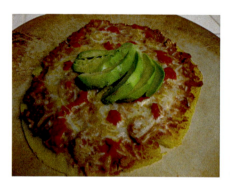

1/2 of a tube of polenta

1/2 of a 15 ounce can of vegetarian refried beans, heated

2-3 Tbsp grated cheese (cheddar or jack or whatever you like)

your favorite smooth salsa

1/2 an avocado, sliced

Preheat oven to 350 degrees. Cut polenta in 1/2 longways and then into 1/4 inch to 1/3 inch wide strips (longways). Arrange slices on a pizza stone or baking sheet. You can cut away the corners to make it into a circle. Spoon heated refried beans onto polenta slices and spread in an even layer. Sprinkle with grated cheese and then add salsa. Bake for 20-25 minutes. Top with avocado. You may need to cut away the edges if they've become too crisp. Omit the cheese to make it dairy-free and cholesterol-free.

Polenta Toppers – Cannellini Beans

Here's another simple, yet flavorful and healthy topping for polenta. Use your own favorite vinaigrette or the one listed here.

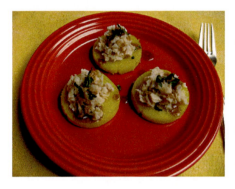

1 tube polenta, cut in 1/4 inch slices

1 15 ounce can cannellini beans, rinsed and drained

Vinaigrette:

3 Tbsp olive oil

1 Tbsp balsamic vinegar

1/4 tsp honey

1/2 tsp Dijon mustard

salt and pepper to taste

Preheat oven to 350. Place polenta slices on baking sheet lined with parchment paper. Bake for 20 minutes. Place cannellini beans on large, flat plate. Mash with back of fork. Mix together all ingredients for vinaigrette in small bowl. When polenta is done, scoop spoonfuls of beans onto each slice and drizzle with dressing.

Polenta Toppers – Chick Pea & Peppers

I used fire-roasted red peppers for this recipe and they have quite a kick! Look for regular roasted peppers if you like less spice.

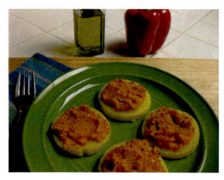

1 tube polenta, cut in 1/4 inch slices

15 ounce can garbanzo beans/chick peas, rinsed and drained

1 small jar of roasted red peppers – you'll just need one section of red pepper, roughly chopped

1 tsp olive oil

1 garlic clove, roughly chopped

1/8 to 1/4 tsp dried oregano

salt and pepper to taste

Preheat oven to 350. Cut polenta into 1/4 inch slices. Place slices on baking sheet lined with parchment paper. Place 1 cup of chick peas, chopped red pepper, olive oil, garlic, oregano and salt and pepper into food processor (I use a mini one). Pulse until well mixed. Spoon about a tablespoon full of mixture onto each polenta slice. Bake 20-25 minutes.

Black Bean Sliders

Black beans are great source of protein and contain no cholesterol. Use a spicy, hot salsa for a little more kick.

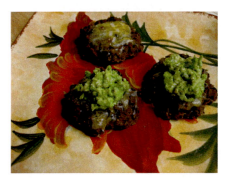

1 15 oz can black beans, rinsed and drained

1 medium or 2 small sweet potatoes, baked, peeled and mashed – about 1/2 cup

1/2 tsp cumin

1/4 tsp chili powder

1 Tbsp your favorite smooth salsa

Optional toppings: cheese, guacamole, mustard, ketchup

Preheat oven to 350. Place beans on plate and use back of fork to press through until softened. Mix beans and mashed sweet potato and add cumin, chili powder and salsa. The mixture will be very wet. Form mixture into small patties – "sliders". Place on baking sheet lined with parchment paper and bake for 20 minutes. If you're adding cheese, bake for another few minutes. Top with your favorite condiments.

Sweet Potato Avocado Roll

Who would have thought you could eat pureed food with chopsticks? Well, I did! I have to say I was very happy that this recipe worked out as well in the kitchen as it did in my head. You can eat it warm or at room temperature.

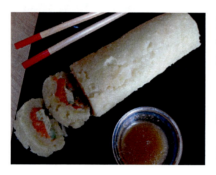

2 small-medium sweet potatoes – baked, cooled, peeled and mashed

1 small-medium yam – baked, cooled, peeled and mashed

1/2 avocado sliced longways

Citrus Dipping Sauce

juice from 1/4 of an orange

1/2 tsp honey

1/2 tsp gluten-free soy sauce

1/8 to 1/4 tsp sesame oil

Bake the sweet potatoes and yams ahead of time and it all comes together pretty quickly. Press the mashed sweet potatoes into a 4 inch by 6 inch rectangle on a piece of parchment paper, with the longer side parallel to you. Add several tablespoons of the yam longways along the center of the rectangle (you may have some left over). Lay the avocado slices on top of the yam. Lift the edge of the parchment paper up and over to form a roll; carefully peeling the sweet potato away from the parchment paper. Press the edges lightly together. Use a spatula to move the roll onto a plate. For the dipping sauce, mix all ingredients well.

Menu suggestion: serve with Carrot Ginger Soup.

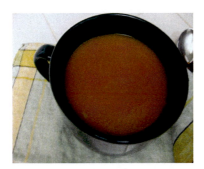

Thai Green Curry

Spice up those chilly winter nights with this curry recipe. Green curry is a blend of green chili, garlic, lemongrass, ginger and a few other spices. The coconut milk keeps it super smooth and the cooked cauliflower makes a nice "holder" for the curry itself.

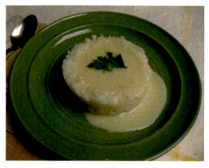

1 cup chopped cauliflower

drizzle of canola oil

2-3 tsp green curry paste

14 oz can coconut milk

1/2 Tbsp brown sugar

1/3 cup vegetable broth

Steam cauliflower 7-8 minutes or until soft enough to be easily mashed with fork. Drain, mash until smooth, adding a drizzle of canola oil. Form into a mound on plate or press into food mold.

While the cauliflower is steaming, stir together coconut milk, curry paste and bring to boil, then reduce to simmer for 5 minutes. Add brown sugar and vegie broth and simmer for 10 more minutes. Serve over cauliflower.

Polentil Strata

"Polentil" comes from a combination of "polenta" and "lentil" (my own invention). I've used them both here for a colorful dish with no fat and lots of protein.

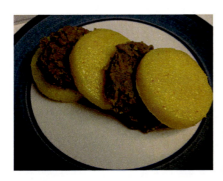

1 tube polenta

1/2 cup dried lentils

1 1/2 – 2 cups water

salt

olive oil

To cook lentils, bring lentils and water to a boil, reduce heat and simmer for 30-40 minutes, adding more water as needed (all of the water will be absorbed). The lentils will break down and become very soft. Add salt to taste (you could also add thyme or oregano) and stir until well blended. This step can be done ahead of time.

Slice polenta into 1/2 inch slices. Place slices in pan heated with a little olive oil over medium heat. Cook for 6-7 minutes per side.

Create layers alternating polenta slices and lentils.

Chick Pea Spinach Patties

A while back, someone asked me "what about the leafy greens?" Since then I've been trying to come up with ways to use spinach in these recipes. Here's one.

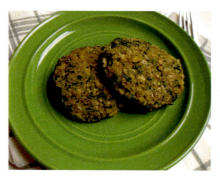

15 oz can chick peas, drained, rinsed and mashed

4 oz frozen chopped spinach, steamed and blended

1/4 cup oats (look for gluten-free oats if you're going gluten-free)

1 1/2 tsp cumin

1 tsp coriander

1/2 tsp garlic powder

1/2 tsp chili powder

1/4 tsp salt

1 Tbsp ground flax mixed with water (to egg consistency)

1 green onion, finely diced

olive or canola oil

Mix all ingredients (except for oil). Using ~1/2 cup of the mixture, form into patties. Place on baking sheet and refrigerate for 30 minutes. Heat small amount of olive or canola oil in non-stick pan or grill pan. Cook patties for 4-5 minutes each side.

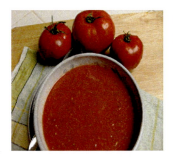

Menu suggestion: serve with Gazpacho Soup.

Spinach Lasagne

Polenta slices stand in for pasta noodles in this version of lasagne, but the combination of marinara sauce, ricotta cheese and spinach makes it taste like the real thing.

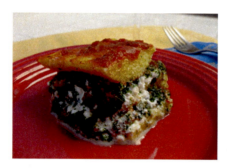

1 tube polenta

4-6 oz frozen, chopped spinach

8 oz ricotta cheese

your favorite marinara sauce (or use recipe listed under Sauces.)

Preheat oven to 350. Steam spinach 5-7 minutes until completely heated through. Add a dash of salt and blend until smooth (you may need to add a little reserved water from steaming the spinach to help it blend more smoothly). Slice polenta longways into 6 equal slices (about 1/4 inch thick). Place 2 slices of polenta side by side in a baking dish (you can line the bottom with parchment paper). Add a layer of ricotta, spinach and marinara sauce. Repeat with another set of layers, ending with a polenta slice and topping it with sauce. Bake for 25-30 minutes.

Vegie Kabobs

I love these purple potatoes – how fun to eat something naturally purple! When cubing the vegies, try to get them all about the same size so they'll cook evenly.

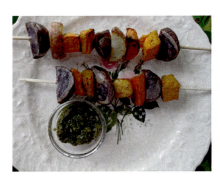

1/2 yam, peeled and cubed

~8 oz butternut squash, peeled and cubed

2-3 small purple potatoes, peeled and cubed

2-3 small red-skinned potatoes, peeled and cubed

olive oil

salt and pepper to taste

Place cubed vegies in a baking dish and lightly drizzle with olive oil, add salt and pepper and mix well. Bake at 400 degrees for 50-55 minutes, or until soft. Allow vegies to cool for a few minutes, then carefully place on wooden skewers, alternating colors. Serve with your favorite dipping sauce.

You can add your favorite pesto sauce, or Garlic and Lemon Dipping Sauce found under Sauces (pesto usually has cheese in it, so use the Garlic and Lemon Dipping Sauce if you're avoiding dairy and cholesterol).

Polenta Pizza Margherita

Pesto sauce substitutes for whole basil leaves in this variation of one of my favorite pizzas.

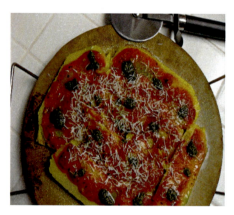

1 tube polenta

your favorite pizza or marinara sauce (or use recipe under Sauces)

your favorite pesto sauce

grated mozzarella cheese (optional)

Pre-heat oven to 350. Slice polenta long-ways into 1/2 inch slices. Arrange polenta slices in a single layer on pizza stone or baking sheet lined with parchment paper. You may want to cut the corners off to make it look like a round "pizza." Add a thin layer of pizza/marinara sauce. Top with drizzles of pesto sauce. Sprinkle with cheese. Bake for 20-25 minutes.

Avocado Chick Pea Salad

Fresh lime juice brightens up all the flavors in this non-traditional "salad."

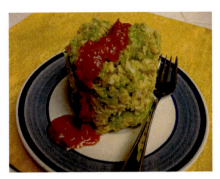

1 avocado, mashed

1/2 of a 15 oz can of chick peas (garbanzo beans), drained and rinsed

juice from one lime

1 garlic clove, minced

dash salt

your favorite (smooth) red salsa

Mix garlic and salt with mashed avocado, set aside. Add chick peas and lime juice to food processor and pulse/blend until smooth. Partially mix avocado and chick pea mixture together. Lightly brush inside of food mold with olive or canola oil. Spoon mixture into mold and lightly press down with spoon. Carefully remove mold. Top with salsa.

Savory Yam Pancakes

A savory version of sweet Yam Pancakes. Feel free to adjust the level of seasoning or use a different combination that suits your taste.

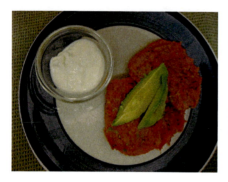

1 16 ounce yam, baked, cooled, peeled and mashed

1/4 cup flour

2 green onions (white and light green parts) thinly sliced

1/4 tsp cumin

1/3 tsp grated ginger

1 Tbsp ground flax mixed with enough water to egg consistency

salt and pepper to taste

avocado or plain yogurt

Mix all ingredients through salt and pepper. Heat a little olive oil in pan over medium heat. Drop batter by 1/4 cup into pan and cook 4-5 minutes per side. Top with avocado (optional). Omit the yogurt and it's dairy-free with no cholesterol. Makes 4 pancakes.

Stuffed Acorn Squash

The seasonings used here can be varied. You can also try thyme, sage, rosemary or cumin instead of nutmeg. Experiment and see what you like.

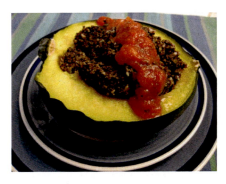

1 acorn squash, cut in 1/2 top to bottom, seeds scooped out

3/4 cup walnuts

3/4 cup mushrooms, chopped

1/2 cup chopped red onion

1/4 tsp nutmeg (or more)

1 Tbsp olive oil

1/4 tsp salt

1/8 tsp pepper

Heat oven to 375. Place squash cut side down in baking dish and fill with 1/2 inch of water. Bake for 45 minutes. In the meantime, use a food processor to blend walnuts into a fine meal. Add mushrooms and red onion, nutmeg, salt and pepper and pulse a few more times until thoroughly mixed. Add olive oil and pulse until mixture seems moist. After the squash has baked 45 minutes, remove from oven and drain water from baking dish. Turn squash halves cut side up and fill with mushroom mixture. Return to oven and bake for another 20 minutes. For a little extra zing, top with your favorite marinara sauce (or see recipe under Sauces).

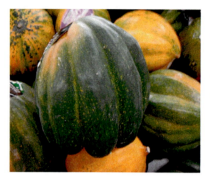

Cutting the squash in half and then leaving it intact to serve as a "bowl" is a great way to enhance the visual appeal of food.

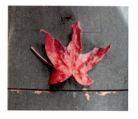

Lentil & Cauliflower Tower

This is fun to build – you can use a metal food mold or just cut both ends off of a 15 oz can. Start cooking the lentils first as they take more time and have to cool a little. Feel free to layer in any order you like.

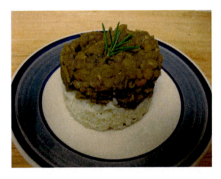

For lentils:

1 cup dry lentils

1 cup vegetable broth

2 cups water

1/2 tsp dried basil

1/4 tsp dried oregano

1/4 tsp dried thyme

1/4 tsp salt

1/8 tsp garlic powder

1/8 tsp pepper

For cauliflower:

2 cups cauliflower cut into small pieces

1 tsp olive oil

salt and pepper to taste

1 Tbsp grated parmesan

 cheese (optional)

Add lentils to water and vegie broth and bring to a boil. Reduce heat and simmer for 20 minutes. Add all seasonings and simmer for 15-20 more minutes, or until lentils are very soft and break down easily. Set aside to cool for 10-15 minutes.

Steam cauliflower for 10-12 minutes. Drain cauliflower and add to bowl with olive oil and salt and pepper. Use back of fork to press through cauliflower until thoroughly blended. Add parmesan cheese and mix well.

Lightly brush inside of mold with olive oil. Add cauliflower to bottom of mold and press down with back of spoon. Add a few spoonfuls of lentils (you will have some left over) as the second layer and press down. Carefully remove mold. Omit the parmesan cheese and it's dairy-free with no cholesterol.

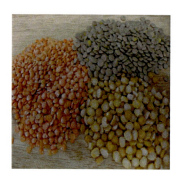

There are several varieties of lentils (yellow, red, green). I used green for this recipe.

Baked Acorn Squash II

I decided to try a different filling for the baked acorn squash. When the squash is baked, it becomes very soft, similar to a mashed potato. If you're watching your sodium intake, check the label on the beans and look for a low-salt version.

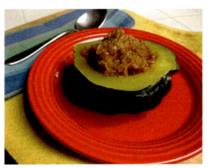

1 acorn squash, cut in 1/2 from top to bottom

1 15 oz can vegetarian baked beans

Preheat oven to 400 degrees. Place squash halves cut-side down in a baking dish and fill with 1/2 inch of water. Bake for 50-60 minutes. Remove water from baking dish and let cool. Heat beans on stovetop to simmer for a few minutes, until heated through. Drain liquid from beans (reserve liquid) and place beans on plate. Use fork to press through beans until completely broken down and smooth. Fill squash halves with beans, pour reserved liquid over top if the beans become too dry.

Black Bean Enchiladas

A great way to satisfy your craving for enchiladas. Serve with Guacamole on top or on the side.

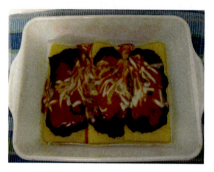

1 tube polenta

1 15 oz can refried black beans (you'll probably have some leftover)

your favorite enchilada sauce

grated cheese

Pre-heat oven to 350.

Warm refried black beans over low heat in saucepan so they will be easier to spread.

Cut ends off of polenta tube (you can top the ends with leftover beans/sauce). Slice polenta long-ways into 1/2 inch slices. Place polenta slices side by side in baking dish lined with parchment paper.

Top each polenta slice with a layer of refried black beans.

Pour enchilada sauce over the top. Sprinkle with grated cheese. Cover and bake for 20 minutes.

Omit the cheese and they're dairy-free and have no cholesterol.

Polenta With Pesto or Marinara Sauce

A wonderful combination of flavors and smells great while it's cooking.

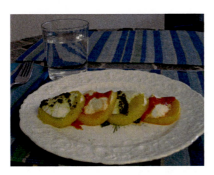

1 tube polenta

Fat-free ricotta cheese

pesto and/or marinara sauce (see the Marinara Sauce recipe under Sauces)

Preheat oven to 350 degrees. Line baking sheet with parchment paper. Cut polenta in 1/4 to 1/3 inch slices and place on lined baking sheet. Top each slice with 1 Tbsp ricotta. Drizzle pesto sauce (a little goes a long way) and/or marinara over each slice. Bake for 20 minutes or until golden.

Menu suggestion: serve with Tomato Basil Soup.

Soups

Fresh vegetables that are in season work best for these soup recipes. If you're not sure if a vegetable is in season, visit your local farmers market to see what the growers are offering that particular week. There you'll also find produce that has been locally grown and is most likely organic.

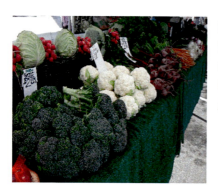

Go to www.localharvest.org to find a farmers market near you and for information on local CSA (Community Supported Agriculture) programs.

Mashed Potato Soup

This is a great way to use any leftover mashed potatoes. Omit the cheese if you're avoiding dairy.

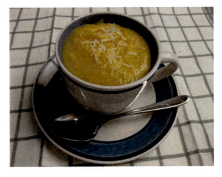

1 large potato, baked, peeled and mashed or ~2 cups of leftover mashed potato

1 small-medium carrot, finely chopped

1/2 small onion, finely chopped

2 garlic cloves, minced

1/2 Tbsp olive oil

salt and pepper to taste

1 cup vegetable broth/water

4 Tbsp shredded cheddar cheese

Heat olive oil in pan over medium heat. Add onions, garlic and carrots and cook for 4-5 minutes, until softened. Add mashed potatoes and cook for another 4-5 minutes. Season with salt and pepper. Add broth or water and stir well. Bring to simmer, cover and simmer for 15-20 minutes. Add 1/2 the cheese and blend (in blender or use immersion blender) until smooth. You may need to add a little more liquid if it's too thick. Top with remaining cheese.

Tomato Basil Soup

Cooler fall weather and a hot bowl of soup go hand in hand. This soup is very simple, just a few ingredients, but very flavorful.

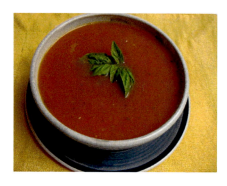

1/2 onion, chopped

1 Tsp olive oil

2 cloves garlic, minced

28 oz can diced tomatoes

32 oz vegetable broth

2-3 Tbsp chopped, fresh basil

salt and pepper to taste

Saute onions in olive oil for several minutes, until translucent. Add garlic and cook 1-2 more minutes. Add tomatoes, broth, basil and salt and pepper. Bring to boil, cover, reduce heat and simmer for 15-20 minutes. Blend until smooth.

Alex's Lentil Soup

This recipe comes all the way from France from my brother Alex – thanks bro! He didn't give me exact measurements for the spices, so I had to estimate. But as always, feel free to adjust seasonings to your own personal taste.

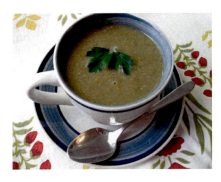

1/2 onion, chopped

olive oil

2-3 carrots, diced

1 small sweet potato, diced

1 cup lentils

5 cups water

14 oz can diced tomatoes

1/2 tsp cumin

1/2 tsp coriander

1/4 tsp paprika or chili powder

1/4 tsp salt

Saute onions in olive oil until soft. Add carrots and sweet potato and cook 4-5 minutes. Add lentils, tomatoes, water and spices. Bring to a boil, reduce heat, cover and simmer for about 45 minutes. Blend soup using a regular or immersion blender.

Gazpacho

Take advantage of fresh tomatoes in season during the summer for this no-cook soup. Just blend all ingredients, chill and serve.

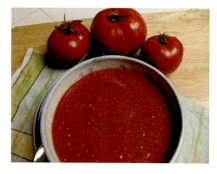

4 large tomatoes, peeled and roughly chopped

1/2 green pepper, chopped

2-3 green onions, chopped

1 cucumber, peeled and chopped

2 cloves garlic

juice from 1 lemon

1/2 to 1 tsp dill

salt and pepper to taste

Blend all ingredients in bowl, serve chilled.

Menu suggestion: serve with Avocado Chick Pea Salad.

Corn Off The Cob Soup

Take advantage of fresh, locally grown corn during the summer. I made this soup from corn I bought at my nearby farmers market. I find a serrated knife works best when cutting the kernels off the cob – stand the corn cob upright in a bowl to catch the kernels.

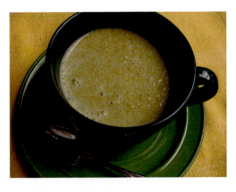

1/2 onion, chopped

1 clove garlic, minced

1Tbsp olive oil

1 1/2 cups vegetable broth

½ cup almond milk

1/2 tsp cumin

salt and pepper to taste

1/4 tsp chili powder

kernels from 2 fresh ears of corn (uncooked), or 2 cups frozen corn, thawed

Heat olive oil over medium heat. Add onions and cook for 3-4 minutes. Add garlic and cook for 1-2 more minutes. Add corn, broth, almond milk and seasonings. Bring to boil, reduce heat, cover and simmer for 10-15 minutes. Blend in batches or use immersion blender to blend soup right in the pot.

Taco Soup

Feel free to adjust the seasonings here; 2 teaspoons of chili powder gives it quite a kick!

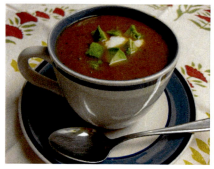

1 medium onion, chopped

2 cloves garlic, minced

2 tsp olive oil

32 oz/4 cups vegetable broth

1 15 oz can black beans, rinsed and drained

1 15 oz can diced tomatoes

1 tsp ground cumin

1 16 oz jar of your favorite salsa

1 small or 1/2 large bell pepper, chopped

1-2 tsp chili powder

Saute onion and garlic in olive oil for several minutes, or until onions are translucent. Add broth, beans, tomatoes, salsa, bell pepper and seasonings. Bring to boil, stirring frequently. Reduce heat, cover and simmer for 10-15 minutes. Blend soup in batches in regular blender or use an immersion blender to blend soup right in the pot. Top with optional garnish: diced avocado and/or plain yogurt.

Carrot Ginger Soup

This soup has a beautiful orange color and a velvety smooth texture. Thank you to Lee Anne for the original recipe which I changed a little bit.

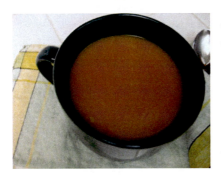

5-6 medium carrots, peeled and thinly sliced

1Tbsp olive oil

1/2 sweet onion, chopped

4 cups vegetable broth

1 Tbsp brown sugar

1 Tbsp grated ginger

salt and pepper to taste

Heat olive oil in pan over medium heat. Add onions and cook 5-7 minutes until translucent. Add ginger and cook 1-2 minutes. Add carrots and brown sugar and cook 5-7 minutes. Add broth, bring to a boil and then reduce heat, cover and simmer for ~20 minutes. Blend soup in batches and return to pot. Add salt and pepper to taste.

Split Pea Soup

A classic from the past. Liquid smoke gives it a wonderful smoky flavor.

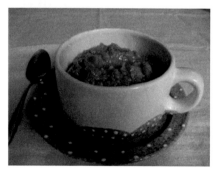

1 cup split peas (green or yellow), rinsed

4 cups water

1/3 cup chopped onion

2-3 carrots, chopped

1-2 tsp no-salt seasoning

2-3 drops liquid smoke – optional

Add peas, carrots and onion to 4 cups water in large pot. Bring to boil, then reduce to simmer and cover. Cook for 45 minutes to an hour, stirring occasionally. Add no-salt seasoning and liquid smoke (if using). If soup is very thick, you can also add more water (1/2 to 1 cup) and simmer for 20 more minutes. Blend if you like a very smooth consistency.

Sides

Here are a few simple and healthy side dishes to enhance the main course. Use no-salt seasonings such as garlic, ginger and cinnamon for a heart-healthy way to enhance flavor.

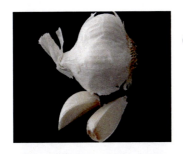 Garlic

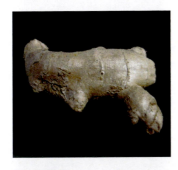 Ginger

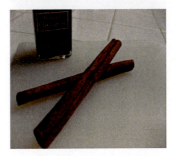 Cinnamon

Tracy's Applesauce

My fellow SLP Tracy has shared this recipe which she makes with her kids. I only altered it a little and cut the portions down to a single serving. You can easily double or triple it. And no cooking required - thanks Tracy!

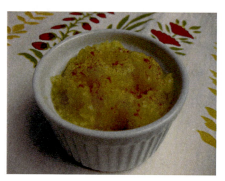

1 large apple, peeled, cored, sliced and cut into 1/2 inch pieces

1/2 tsp honey

dash cinnamon

1/2 tsp water

Add all ingredients to a food processor and pulse several times until smooth. You can always add more water if it's too thick or more cinnamon (or other seasonings) to your taste. Spoon into serving dish and top with a little more cinnamon.

Baked Yam

Yams are naturally sweet and flavorful so they really don't need any seasoning (personally, I like them plain), but if you must, keep it minimal.

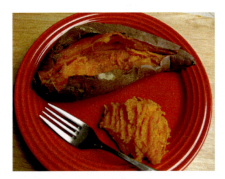
1 yam

Pre-heat oven to 400 degrees. Poke holes all over the yam with a fork. Bake for 40-50 minutes. Let cool slightly. Slice down the middle and eat right out of the shell or scoop out onto plate.

Menu suggestion: serve with Polentil Strata.

Creamed Spinach

Using coconut milk keeps this recipe dairy-free with no cholesterol. A great way to get your greens!

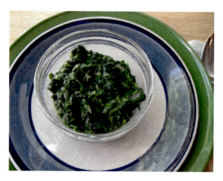

1 Tbsp chopped onion

1 Tbsp olive oil

1 cup frozen, chopped spinach

light dusting of nutmeg

salt and pepper to taste

1 Tbsp coconut milk, plus a little more for blending

Saute onions in olive oil over medium heat for several minutes until translucent. Add spinach and cook for 7-8 minutes. Add salt, pepper, nutmeg and coconut milk and cook for 2-3 minutes until heated through. Remove from heat and blend until smooth, adding 1-2 more tablespoons of coconut milk if needed.

Guacamole

Guacamole complements many foods, not just Mexican dishes.

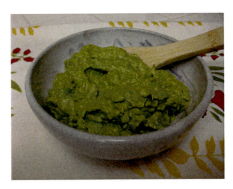

2 ripe avocados

2 Tbsp (or more) your favorite salsa (smooth, not chunky)

pinch salt

pinch cumin (or to taste)

Cut avocados in 1/2 and carefully remove seed. Scoop out avocado onto plate. Use back of fork to press through avocado until smooth. Transfer to bowl. Add salsa, salt and cumin and mix well.

Menu suggestion: serve with Black Bean Enchiladas, Taco Soup or Polenta Tostada.

Garlic Mashed Potatoes

Garlic adds a boost of flavor to otherwise bland potatoes. You can also experiment with different types of potatoes.

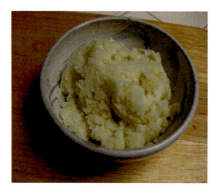

1 russet potato, peeled and cut into 1 inch cubes

1-2 cloves of garlic, minced or pushed through a garlic press

1/4 cup almond milk or vegetable broth

1/2 Tbsp olive oil

salt and pepper to taste

Place potato cubes in pot and fill with enough water to cover. Bring to boil and cook for 10-12 minutes (or until a fork easily presses through). Drain potatoes and place in bowl. Add garlic, almond milk or vegie broth and salt and pepper and olive oil. Mash with potato masher or pastry blender to desired consistency, adding more liquid as needed.

On the Sweet Side

You can indulge your sweet tooth without loading up on sugar. Fresh fruit that is ripe and at its peak is naturally quite sweet. Also try pure maple syrup, honey or agave nectar. A little goes a long way for these natural sweeteners.

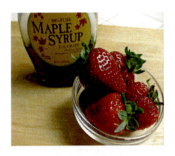

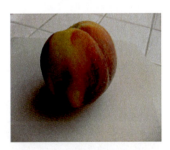

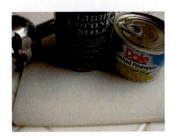

Tiramisu

Tirami su means "pick me up" and a few bites will definitely lift your troubles away. I've made a few changes to this classic Italian dessert, but I think the basic flavors are intact. It's made with mascarpone cheese which is a sweet, creamy cheese, and is very rich (a little goes a long way).

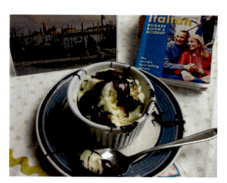

4 ounces mascarpone cheese

2 tsp honey

2 Tbsp chocolate chips, melted

your favorite coffee

Mix mascarpone cheese and honey well and spoon into dessert dish. Drizzle melted chocolate over the top, then a little bit of your favorite coffee.

Go Green Vegie Pops

This is a variation on another recipe (Tropical Freeze). Adding a handful of spinach (kale would probably work too, I used spinach here) ups the nutritional value and they still taste great! A refreshing way to end a warm summer evening.

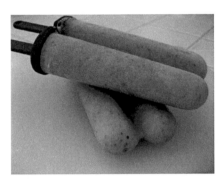

handful of baby spinach (rinsed)

1 cup crushed pineapple (add the juice, too)

3/4 cup coconut milk

2-3 tsp agave or honey

juice from 1/2 lime

Blend all ingredients and pour into popsicle molds. Freeze for 4 hours or over night. Thaw slightly or run popsicle molds under warm water to remove. Makes 4 popsicles.

Peach Crumble

Take advantage of summer fruit that is in season. Shop at your local farmers market for locally grown fruit that has been recently picked.

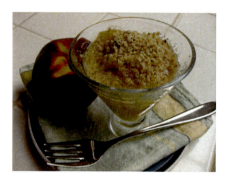

1 very ripe peach, peeled, seed removed

1-2 Tbsp walnuts

dash cinnamon

Slice peach and place slices in small saucepan over low heat. Heat for 3-4 minutes, stirring frequently. Pour peach slices onto plate and use fork to press through (at this point you can blend them for a smoother texture). Place peach puree into dessert dish. Pulse walnuts and cinnamon in food processor until they are very finely ground. Sprinkle over peach puree.

Tropical Freeze

This refreshing dessert will definitely help beat the heat on a hot summer day. And it's dairy-free!

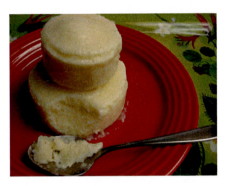

1 cup crushed pineapple (in pineapple juice)

1/2 cup coconut milk

1 tsp agave nectar

Blend all ingredients until very smooth and pour into popsicle molds, ice cube trays, mugs or food molds. Freeze for 4 hours or overnight. Thaw slightly to unmold.

Menu suggestion: serve after eating anything hot and spicy.

Sauces

Citrus Dipping Sauce

- juice from 1/4 of an orange
- 1/2 tsp honey
- 1/2 tsp gluten-free soy sauce
- 1/8 to 1/4 tsp sesame oil

Mix all ingredients.

Ginger Peanut Dipping Sauce

- 1/4 cup creamy peanut butter
- 1 tsp garlic, minced
- 3 Tbsp fresh ginger, minced
- 2 Tbsp brown sugar
- 2 Tbsp low sodium soy sauce

Whisk together all ingredients and 1/3 cup warm water.

Yogurt Dipping Sauce

- 1/2 cup plain yogurt
- 1/2 Tbsp lemon juice
- 1/2 Tbsp lemon zest
- 1/4 Tbsp ground cumin
- salt and pepper to taste

Combine all ingredients in serving bowl.

Garlic Lemon Dipping Sauce

- 1-2 medium cloves garlic, minced
- 1/4 tsp salt
- 2 Tbsp chopped parsley
- pinch dried oregano
- pinch dried basil
- pinch pepper
- juice from 1/2 lemon
- 1/4 cup olive oil

In a small bowl, use the back of a spoon to press the garlic into the salt until mixed. Add parsley, oregano, basil and pepper and mix well. Stir in lemon juice and olive oil.

Marinara Sauce

- 1 Tbsp olive oil
- 1/3 cup chopped onion
- 1-2 cloves garlic, minced
- 1 15 oz can whole tomatoes
- several leaves of fresh basil or 1 tsp dried basil
- 1/2 tsp dried oregano
- salt to taste

Heat olive oil in pan over medium heat. Add onions and cook for several minutes or until translucent. Add garlic and cook for one more minute. Blend whole tomatoes in blender until smooth and add to onion mixture. Add basil, oregano and salt. Bring to simmer and simmer for 30-40 minutes.

Made in the USA
Lexington, KY
17 October 2014